IZZY'S EATING PLAN

A SIMPLE AND HEALTHY WAY TO REACH YOUR WEIGHT LOSS GOAL AND MAINTAIN IT FOR THE REST OF YOUR LIFE.

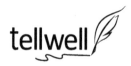

Tellwell Talent
www.tellwell.ca

ISBN
978-1-77302-969-6 (Paperback)
978-1-77302-970-2 (eBook)

TABLE OF CONTENTS

INTRODUCTION:
BE GOOD TO YOURSELF 1

PREFACE:
JOANNE SMITH 5

CHAPTER 1
OWNERSHIP:
CARDS ARE IN YOUR HANDS 7

CHAPTER 2
PLANNING AND LEARNING:
LET'S GET STARTED! 13

CHAPTER 3
MAKING BETTER CHOICES AND
LOOKING OUT FOR YOU! 23

CHAPTER 4
LIFESTYLE CHOICES – GET OUTSIDE! 37

CHAPTER 5
IZZY'S EATING PLAN:
SO EXCITED TO SHARE! 41

CHAPTER 6
FINDING NEW WAYS:
LOOKING AT FOOD DIFFERENTLY 63

CHAPTER 7
AN APPLE A DAY 67

ACKNOWLEDGEMENTS 71

INTRODUCTION: BE GOOD TO YOURSELF

My name is Izzy Camilleri. I'm a very busy fashion designer, entrepreneur and mom. My days are always hectic, whether I'm working on a new fashion collection, costumes for movies and television or creating pieces for iconic A-list celebrities. Since 1984, my fashion design work has focused on making people look awesome and feel great wearing the clothes created for them.

A few years ago, I was inspired with a new focus... an area in my life that had been neglected for way too long. My own health, well-being and weight. I looked in the mirror and decided it was time to concentrate on me.

With my busy schedule, taking care of myself became secondary to everything else. When it came to meal planning for myself and my family, the decisions were often overwhelming. From what to prepare that is easy and quick, to fast food options when there is no time to cook, to eating out, holidays... all while trying to keep everyone happy and satisfied. Not knowing how to work my way through it all without gaining weight seemed like a losing battle.

In my late 40's, I started to notice the effects, and really felt the burden of the extra weight I had been carrying for most of my life. I was always aware of my extra weight, but wasn't very good at doing anything about it. I had tried many diets that would get me to a healthier weight, but the results never lasted. Once I was off the diet, the weight always came back... always.

When I finally made the decision to focus on myself and make a true commitment to improve my health, I thought about the weight-loss plans I had tried in the past. There were many... some were great for a time, others were impossible to stick to. Nonetheless, through trial and error, and my own R&D, I've learned a lot. Most importantly, I learned about the actual cause of my weight gain, which in turn, changed how I look at food, and how I eat today.

My journey to better health became inspiring. People started to notice the changes. I wanted to share my experiences with everyone I spoke to. I felt so great and wanted everyone else to feel great too! What I've learned is such a simple concept... one that's realistic and attainable, no matter where you are in life. We all make food choices everyday, but often without thinking about the impact on our bodies. After reading my book, you'll know how to make informed food choices with everyday foods. Izzy's Eating Plan works whether or not you choose to include animal proteins in your diet, or follow a vegetarian or vegan diet. You'll develop better eating habits that will result in weight loss at a healthy and realistic pace, while improving your overall well-being. You'll feel the importance to put yourself first and begin your own journey for improved health.

While still attending to the needs of the fashion world, my personal focus revolves around inner beauty, good health and well-being.

Take control now... for today and all of your tomorrows.

PREFACE:
JOANNE SMITH

It has been an honour getting to know internationally acclaimed fashion designer Izzy Camilleri. First, as someone whose style of clothing I adored, to becoming good friends, to being fortunate enough to brandish some of her astonishing outfits at several of her stunning fashion shows.

Izzy is nothing short of a creative genius. But, as with so many of us with busy lives, watching what she ate became an afterthought. Over the years, she began to feel her fast-paced lifestyle and eating habits take their toll on her.

As a nutritionist, I work with a myriad of clients who have vastly different agendas and goals that they wish to achieve and a variety of demands on their time. For many of my clients changing their eating habits is a complete lifestyle change that can seem overwhelming. In this information age, we are inundated, often by conflicting facts, on what, how, where, when, and why to eat certain foods.

The simple fact is – the key to living well is eating well. If you can optimize your health through a healthy diet you can live your life to its fullest potential.

In Izzy's Eating Plan, Izzy has created well-balanced guidelines that are simple and easy to understand and more than anything - simple to follow.

For someone accustomed to creating outfits to make people look and feel beautiful, Izzy has designed another masterpiece or pièce de résistance with her new book Izzy's Eating Plan that will help you look and feel the way you want to live your life to the fullest.

Joanne Smith B.A., BRT, CNP
Nutritionist

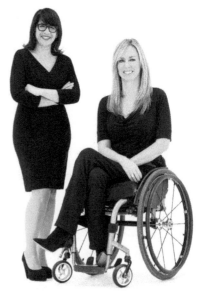

CHAPTER 1

OWNERSHIP:
CARDS ARE IN YOUR HANDS

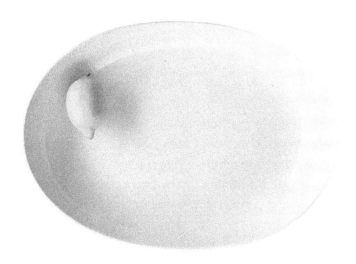

OWNERSHIP: CARDS ARE IN YOUR HANDS

Our bodies are our personal temples. We need to respect and take care of them as best we can every day and at every meal. Treating our bodies with respect includes taking ownership of our actions, as well as being responsible for the outcome of these actions. Yes, this includes taking responsibility for what and why we eat, as well as how we eat it. If you are overweight, think about your past and present eating habits... probably not much has changed over the years. It's that simple – if you continue to make the same food choices, you'll continue to carry extra weight. Our bodies are a direct result of our actions, good or bad. Continuing any bad habit can be fatal. Over eating, smoking, alcohol or drug use (legal or illegal) violates our bodies, breaking them down, allowing for health issues to develop that can become extremely damaging or irreversible. Creating and continuing good habits will lead to improved, overall health and a feeling of self-accomplishment. Once you realize this and are ready to take TRUE ownership, you can move forward and take control of your life and your weight, which will allow for balance and a healthier new you. Making this decision to take hold of your own situation, to put yourself and your health first is the best thing you can do for yourself, your body and your future.

Growing up, many of us were not given the right guidance or education around food. We weren't taught that the food choices we make affect our weight, or that when counting calories, you also need to consider the source of the calories. Consider the term "malnourished". I always understood this to mean that someone was underweight, not getting enough food or the right nutrients. Although this is true, it can also refer to someone who is overweight. Being malnourished is simply a lack of proper nutrition, whether you are underweight or overweight. Perhaps, like myself, you have been overweight since childhood. You've always seen yourself in this way and haven't thought much more about it, or didn't think you could change it. I didn't see myself as being malnourished or in poor health, but I was. The proof was in my weight. When we carry extra weight, we put stress on our bodies, and organs. Over time, our bones and joints begin to wear down bearing this extra weight. We are at greater risk of health issues developing, such as cardiovascular disease and type 2 diabetes, which can turn into a rollercoaster of physical and emotional issues. We just don't function properly. Take comfort in the fact that you CAN see yourself differently. You CAN take charge of your present and your future. Do not allow the past to hold you back. I did just this. I wanted to see myself differently, so I took ownership of my actions and responsibility for my weight. My weight that was created by me. I knew that I needed to change my life long bad eating habits so that I could be a healthier me, for my present and my future.

For the first time, after taking ownership, my weight loss became inspirational and thought provoking. By following a simple way of eating, I was able to lose the weight, by myself. I came to realize just how many diet plans are difficult to follow and simply not realistic.

I, like many people, have tried fad diets or even joined diet clinics to help with my weight issues. When I reflect now on those diets, I feel it was a false sense of weight loss. Like it wasn't 'me' who lost the weight, but the program that made my body lose the weight, AND in an unnatural and unrealistic way. I followed these diets, and I was responsible for making them work, but I was handing myself over to the program. I could not make the weight loss happen on my own. These fad diets either worked too fast, were too ridged or impossible to sustain over time, with or without being on a program.

Although you do lose the weight from such diets, the expectations are often too high or unhealthy. It's not healthy to lose 10-16 pounds in one month as one of the diet plans I was on guaranteed. I also came to learn that many people experience major health issues after going on these types of diets. I, myself, started to lose my hair during one weight loss program I was on. When I expressed concern and asked about it, I was told at the diet clinic, that it was because my body was 'in stress' from the rapid weight loss. They told me to increase my vitamin intake and didn't seem to be surprised or worried about it. I, of course was freaking out... I was losing my hair!!! It took years for my thinning hair to fill back out and feel normal again. And hair loss isn't the only negative side effect when dropping pounds too quickly. Our skin is also affected. It simply can't keep up to such rapid weight loss. It tends to sag and lose elasticity, causing a gaunt or ill look. I'm sure the gaunt look is not what we are going for. Obviously, we shouldn't be putting our bodies into stress or danger when trying to lose weight.

Intense, or fad diets may get us to our goal weight, but often, we're left feeling deprived. We miss the foods that were restricted or 'off-limits' and may 'reward' ourselves for our weight loss by having these 'treats' again. In return, you guessed it, the weight comes back and sometimes more than was lost. Going back to old eating habits will get you back to where you started. Such a simple statement that makes so much sense, and has been proven time and time again. Our bodies are only reacting to our actions, and in this case, our food choices. If we don't commit to change, then nothing will change. If we understand why we carried extra weight in the first place, and have the knowledge and understanding of how the weight was both gained and lost, we will have an easier time committing to change. Knowing that what and how we are eating has a direct impact on our weight will help us to make better, healthier choices. Thinking about what and how we are eating throughout the entire day at every meal, will help maintain a healthy weight and body, even after your goal is reached.

One of the things about my eating plan that I LOVE, is that I really did lose the weight on my own. I didn't have to pay high fees to follow a program, visit a clinic, take any pills, injections or supplements. No calorie counting, weighing or purchasing special foods. All the foods are from my local grocery store. Nothing fancy, just simple everyday stuff. I did it on my own terms giving myself time to lose the weight without any unrealistic or unhealthy expectations. It was manageable and continues to be. If I can do it, you can do it too.

Believe in yourself. I believe in you.

CHAPTER 2

PLANNING AND LEARNING: LET'S GET STARTED!

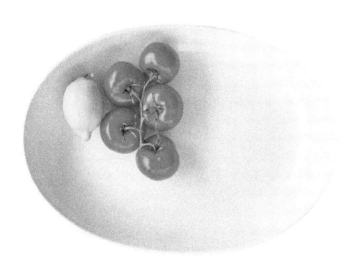

PLANNING AND LEARNING: LET'S GET STARTED!

You've decided to take ownership of your health and body weight. Now you can take control, no longer allowing your weight and food choices to control you.

Take some time to decide on how much weight you'd like to lose. Included here is a chart on advised body weight pending gender, height and body frame. This chart is only a guide for you to find your optimal weight. There will be a point within the advised weight range where you feel great and healthy... around that 'feeling great' number is the ideal weight you should be.

AVERAGE WEIGHT FOR ADULT MALES

HEIGHT		SMALL FRAME		MEDIUM FRAME		LARGE FRAME	
FEET	METERS	POUNDS	KILOS	POUNDS	KILOS	POUNDS	KILOS
5'	1.52	112-117	50-53	120-125	54-56	129-134	58-60
5'1"	1.55	115-120	52-54	123-128	55-58	131-136	59-61
5'2"	1.57	118-123	53-55	126-131	57-59	133-138	60-62
5'3"	1.60	121-126	54-57	129-134	58-60	135-140	61-63
5'4"	1.63	124-129	56-58	132-137	59-62	141-146	64-66
5'5"	1.65	128-133	58-60	137-142	62-64	145-150	65-68
5'6"	1.68	132-137	59-62	140-145	63-65	148-153	67-69
5'7"	1.70	136-141	61-64	143-148	64-67	153-158	69-71
5'8"	1.73	139-141	63-65	148-153	67-69	157-162	71-73
5'9"	1.75	143-148	64-67	152-157	69-71	161-166	73-75
5'10"	1.78	148-153	67-69	157-162	71-73	166-171	75-77
5'11"	1.80	151-156	68-70	160-165	72-74	170-175	77-79
6'	1.83	156-161	70-73	165-170	74-77	175-180	79-81
6'1"	1.85	161-166	73-75	170-175	77-79	180-185	81-84
6'2"	1.88	167-172	75-78	175-180	79-81	185-190	84-86
6'3"	1.91	172-177	78-80	180-185	81-84	190-195	86-88
6'4"	1.93	177-182	80-82	185-190	84-86	195-200	88-90

AVERAGE WEIGHT FOR ADULT FEMALES

HEIGHT		SMALL FRAME		MEDIUM FRAME		LARGE FRAME	
FEET	METERS	POUNDS	KILOS	POUNDS	KILOS	POUNDS	KILOS
4'10"	1.47	103-108	46-49	110-115	49-52	118-123	53-55
4'11"	1.50	105-110	47-50	112-117	50-53	120-125	54-56
5'0"	1.52	107-112	48-51	114-119	51-54	122-127	55-57
5'1"	1.55	109-114	49-52	116-121	52-54	124-129	56-58
5'2"	1.57	112-117	50-53	119-124	54-56	127-132	57-59
5'3"	1.60	115-120	52-54	122-127	55-57	130-135	59-61
5'4"	1.63	118-123	53-55	126-131	57-59	134-139	60-63
5'5"	1.65	121-126	54-57	129-134	58-60	137-142	62-64
5'6"	1.68	125-130	56-59	133-138	60-62	142-147	64-66
5'7"	1.70	129-134	58-60	137-142	62-64	146-151	66-68
5'8"	1.73	132-137	59-62	140-145	63-65	149-154	67-69
5'9"	1.75	136-141	61-64	144-149	65-67	153-158	69-71
5'10"	1.78	139-144	63-65	148-153	67-69	157-162	71-73
5'11"	1.80	142-147	64-66	151-156	68-70	160-165	72-74
6'0"	1.83	145-150	65-68	155-160	70-72	163-168	74-76
6'1"	1.85	148-153	67-69	158-163	71-74	166-171	75-77
6'2"	1.88	151-156	68-70	161-166	73-75	169-174	76-79

Next, you can estimate how much time it will take to reach your goal.

On my eating plan, you can realistically lose one to two pounds per week. Use this to calculate your estimated completion date. Planning this out, having a completion date in mind, is a great way to keep you on track. Remember, it took your body time to gain weight, so give your body the time to lose it. Don't be in a rush. Losing one to two pounds a week may not seem like a lot, but it is a healthy amount to lose. Any more than this does not allow your body the time to make the necessary internal adjustments, and could lead to loss of precious muscle instead of loss of fat. Diet plans promoting excessive, rapid weight loss are not ones to consider.

When working out your weight loss goals, it's important to consider timing. There will always be situations or special events that come up from time to time that may impede your schedule. Keep this in mind, and be flexible with your goal completion date, knowing that there will be circumstances beyond your control.

There will be other challenges too, throughout your weight loss journey, that will make you glad you've given yourself some extra time to reach your goal. Let's discuss some of these. Water retention and the initial flush. This is often noticed right out of the gate. You instantly drop pounds and feel great about your progress! The challenge? Some time passes and your progress slows down. Don't worry, this happens to everyone. Because you are now making healthier food choices, you are consuming less foods that cause your body to retain fluids (i.e. sodium, refined carbohydrates), and you are seeing the results of the initial flush. Knowing this is normal, you stay on track with the eating plan and continue to drop pounds. Great! After some more time passes, we find ourselves hitting the next challenge. Again, it seems the scale is stuck, and you've been so careful, religiously sticking to your new way of eating. Don't get discouraged! This also happens to everyone, and is commonly known as a 'plateau'. Perhaps you've experienced this with past diets and know that it is only temporary. This is another adjustment period for your body. It is learning to adapt to your weight loss and new way of eating. Your body needs this time, so don't let the plateaus get the best of you! They will happen, but they will end too. What's important is that you are feeding your body healthy foods and creating better eating habits. Whether you have 10 pounds to lose or 100, you WILL get there. I believe in you! Give your body and mind all the time it needs to adjust and reach your goal. Stay on track, keep positive and you will be stronger for it!

Eating out and going to parties are a way of life for some people. Others, it's an occasional event. Regardless, when you're trying to watch what you eat, someone else's menu can seem like a road block. We've all been there and know there aren't always healthy options available, but you've gotta eat! In the past, if I ate poorly at a function or restaurant while on a weight loss program, I would feel I had completely spoiled my diet. I felt like I had literally 'fallen off the wagon' and there was no point continuing. It was always so devastating for me. Now, I have learned to look at these situations differently. We all deserve to have a good time now and then, so when I'm invited to a party, I enjoy myself! I make the best food choices I can, have a treat if I feel inclined, and go right back to my eating plan the very next meal. The same goes for when I'm eating at a restaurant. I look at the menu for the best food options closest to my eating plan, choosing lighter meals over heavy, rich foods. When I am finished, I don't feel sluggish, or that I've eaten too much, and my weight loss is not negatively affected. No harm done.

When you reach the halfway point of your completion date, I encourage you to take a break. Yup, take a break. I suggest two to four weeks. It may sound counter-productive, but it isn't. This is not a race, and your target completion date is not set in stone. During this break is when you will follow the maintenance part of my eating plan (explained in Chapter 5), and really get used to your new way of eating. It should start to feel like second nature, requiring little thought about the food choices you make. Remember, you still need to be accountable for what you are eating, and stay true to yourself. Your new awareness and understanding around food will become common practice. Your end goal is to not go back to the way you ate before. Your goal is to put your health, body and future first by creating and maintaining better, healthier eating habits.

Below are a couple of examples you can use to determine your estimated completion date, based on losing one to two pounds per week:

20lbs @ 2lbs loss per week = 10 weeks ÷ 4 (4 weeks per month) = 2.5 months
20lbs @ 1.5lbs loss per week = 13 weeks ÷ 4 = 3 months
20lbs @ 1lb loss per week = 20 weeks ÷ 4 = 5 months

Let's do the same for a 50 pound weight loss:

50lbs @ 2lbs loss per week = 25 weeks ÷ 4 = 6 months
50lbs @ 1.5lbs loss per week = 33 weeks ÷ 4 = 8 months
50lbs @ 1lb loss per week = 50 weeks ÷ 4 = 12.5 months

Therefore, a healthy 20lb weight loss can take anywhere from 2.5-5 months. A healthy 50lb weight loss can take anywhere from 6-12.5 months. This time range absorbs expected obstacles (plateaus, halfway point break, special events, etc.) that may hinder weight loss.

During my weight loss, out of curiosity, I weighed myself every morning after I woke up. Even though I was following my eating plan religiously, my weight fluctuated daily by 0-3 pounds. Many diet plans do not encourage weighing yourself daily for this reason - it can be discouraging to see your weight going up when you expect it to go down. However, I learned that this is completely normal and decided to record my results. The main reason for this variation in weight is water retention, which has many contributing factors - sodium or carbohydrate intake, alcohol consumption, hormone changes, natural bodily functions, etc. What I noticed was a constant increase or decrease for a few days before a pound was completely lost. Since I knew I was not eating badly, I found this intriguing rather than discouraging. You can chart your weight once a week or daily, as a tool, to help you see where you are and stay on track. Be patient and give your body the time it naturally needs to reach your goal.

UNDERSTANDING HOW
WE GAIN WEIGHT:

WEIGHT GAIN:

During the process of digestion, after consuming unhealthy, refined, high glycemic carbohydrate foods, large amounts of sugar enter our blood stream quickly. In response, the pancreas releases excess insulin to try and move these large amounts of sugar into our cells. If we are consistently eating sugar laden foods resulting in high blood sugar and insulin levels, our cells may stop responding to the insulin, thus sugar stays in our blood stream. These sugars will then be stored as fat and may also contribute to the development of type 2 diabetes.

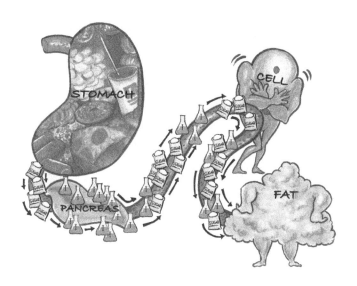

WEIGHT LOSS:

During the process of digestion, after consuming healthy complex carbohydrate foods (high fibre foods), sugars from these foods slowly enter the blood stream. The hormone insulin is then released more gradually from our pancreas to help move sugars from our blood, into our cells so they can be utilized as energy. Eating a consistent healthy well balanced diet will result in maintaining a healthy weight.

With Izzy's Eating Plan, we are consuming healthy high fibre, nutrient dense foods that help keep blood sugar and insulin levels balanced. When our cells have used up the energy provided through the foods we've eaten following the plan, they will use up fat reserves for more required energy, this is when weight loss occurs.

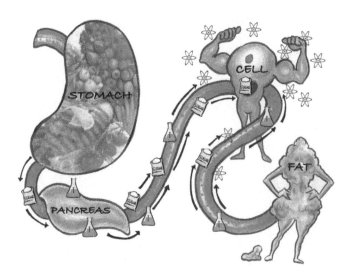

CHAPTER 3

MAKING BETTER CHOICES
AND LOOKING OUT FOR YOU!

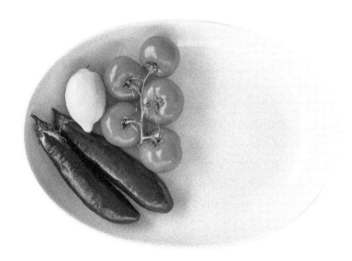

MAKING BETTER CHOICES AND LOOKING OUT FOR YOU!

Look at food differently. Food is fuel for your body. Just as a car needs fuel to run, your body needs food to function. If you give a car bad fuel, it runs poorly. If you let the car run out of fuel, it stops running all together. Your body is the same. Food is fuel. While eating for pleasure, we also need to eat with intention and purpose. We need to keep our bodies filled with good fuel. Skipping meals should not enter our minds, or be thought of as a way to lose a few pounds. It actually has the opposite effect. When we deprive ourselves of food, our bodies hold on to its fat reserves and may begin to break down healthy muscle tissue. There are other negative side effects too. Headaches, irritability, light-headedness and feeling weak are just a few. This is not what we want. We want to keep our bodies fueled with healthy foods to keep the weight dropping.

Choose foods that are fresh and whole. Raw fruits and vegetables and whole grains contain more fibre and nutrients than processed or canned foods respectively, making them more filling. When possible, support your local farmers by shopping at farmer's markets and choosing organically grown produce. Adding these fresh, raw, whole grain foods to every meal are excellent ways to increase fibre. You will eat less because you will feel full longer and you will give your body the nutrients it needs for a good cleanse and workout while improving your digestive health.

Have healthy snacks on hand. This is especially important when introducing new eating habits. You will be eating differently than you're used to, and you may feel hungry for the first few days while your body adjusts. When you feel hungry, start with a glass of water. Often times, thirst is mistaken for hunger. If you still don't feel completely satisfied, by all means, have a healthy snack. If you're used to reaching for junk food, this is the time we need to remember that junk food is just that... JUNK! Was there ever a time you had only one potato chip? Not for me... one always lead to two... and then another, and then a handful. Instead of testing our strength and will power, it is best to resist junk food altogether. Out of sight, out of mind and out of reach. By having your home stocked with healthy snacks, you won't be tempted to eat something you shouldn't out of convenience or habit.

Drink lots of water. I know this can be a challenge because it is for me. I don't like to drink cold water, so I have mine at room temperature. Sometimes I add some lemon for a bit of flavour. If it still feels like a chore to drink water, simply try to drink more fluids. Herbal teas and diluted juices are a good option, and green tea is proven to promote weight loss. Every part of our body needs to be hydrated, and water is the best option. The more water you drink, the more your body will crave it.

Many people are not aware that one of the ways fat leaves our bodies is through our fluids. Or that our body requires water in order for our cells to make use of the nutrients we feed it. These two points will hopefully help encourage you to drink more water, knowing it's a vehicle for fat to exit our body, and it's vital for nutrient absorption.

When I started my new way of eating, I became more curious about foods and their benefits. I did some digging and learned that different foods affected my body in different ways. I wanted to know more. I wanted to use foods to my advantage and target my own areas for improvement. I no longer wanted to eat on 'auto-pilot' as so many of us do. I wanted to feed my body well and do it consciously.

First, I wanted a fresh start. A cleanse was in order, but I had read that juice cleanses were very hard on your liver. I did not want to put my body in any danger. How else could I achieve this? I did some research to find foods that are natural cleansers. I found that many of these were in my eating plan and started including these in my meals and snacks everyday. I was cleansing as I was digesting, and noticing the results! This sparked my curiosity even further.

Listed here are foods that are natural cleansers:

- Apples
- Asparagus
- Avocado
- Beets
- Broccoli, Cauliflower, Cabbage, Brussels Sprouts
- Dark Berries
- Kale
- Legumes
- Lemon
- Spinach

Natural cleansers will improve all aspects of your body and overall health... but why stop there? I continued my research to find foods that would benefit my heart, brain, bones, skin and hair. Encouraged by what I was finding, I continued to include these foods daily. Over time, I noticed visible improvements while losing weight at the same time! One, in particular, went unnoticed by me until I started receiving compliments. My skin looked great and others were noticing! I wasn't aware of my new fresh glow, and had never gotten compliments on my skin before... I was a bit confused. I needed to find out why I was suddenly so radiant, so I spoke to a nutritionist about it. I learned that my skin was literally glowing! Because I was regularly eating foods that are natural cleansers, my liver was functioning at its absolute best, ridding my body of toxins that normally exit through our skin. Without these toxins in my body, my skin no longer looked dull or greasy, but looked healthy and luminous. For the first time in a long time, I liked what I saw in the mirror, and felt better about myself and the way I looked.

Below are my lists of foods that benefit different areas of your body. Use these lists to determine how you can best take advantage of food, and target your body for specific improvements. Let the compliments roll in and smile at your reflection!

Foods that will benefit your heart:

- Almonds and Walnuts
- Beans (black or navy)
- Berries
- Brown Rice
- Fish (cold water fish such as salmon, mackerel, trout, sardines)
- Garlic
- Mushrooms
- Oatmeal
- Spinach
- Tomatoes

Foods that will benefit your bones:

- Almonds
- Broccoli
- Cheese
- Green Leafy Vegetables
- Legumes
- Parsley
- Salmon (with bones)
- Sardines (with bones)
- Sesame Seeds
- Unsweetened Greek Yogurt

Foods that will benefit your brain:

- Blueberries
- Dark Chocolate (70% cocoa or more)
- Eggs
- Kale
- Legumes and Lentils
- Quinoa
- Salmon
- Unsweetened Greek Yogurt
- Walnuts
- Whole Grains

Foods that will benefit your skin:

- Beets
- Berries
- Green Tea
- Kale
- Oatmeal
- Olives/Olive Oil
- Pumpkin Seeds
- Sweet Potatoes
- Tomatoes
- Unsweetened Greek Yogurt

Foods that will benefit your hair:

- Chicken
- Eggs
- Legumes
- Lentils
- Oatmeal
- Salmon
- Sweet Potatoes
- Tangerines
- Walnuts and Almonds
- Whole Grains

Did you know that there are foods that take more energy to digest than the calories they contain? These foods are great to eat during your weight loss as they give your insides a workout and help contribute to your weight loss goal.

Listed below are foods that take more energy to burn than the calories they contain:

- Almonds
- Apples
- Avocados
- Beans
- Berries
- Broccoli, Cauliflower, Cabbage, Brussels Sprouts
- Brown Rice
- Celery
- Eggs
- Green Tea
- Leafy Greens/Spinach
- Lean Beef/Chicken Breast/Fish (salmon, halibut, trout, tilapia)

Here are some helpful suggestions to keep in mind as you work toward your goal:

- Eat 5 times a day. 3 full meals and 2 snacks following Izzy's Eating Plan.
- Drink water. Aim for 6-8 8 oz. glasses daily.
- Reduce your dairy intake, as it may act as an inflammatory. For example switch to black coffee or clear tea.
- Have 5-10 servings of vegetables and 1-2 servings of fruits per day. Support local farmer's markets. Purchase farm fresh, organically grown produce whenever possible.
- Be fully aware of what you are eating and make each meal count.
- Try to include a protein at every main meal.
- Including raw and high fibre foods is a great way to give your body a workout, stay full longer and help to cleanse your insides too!
- When deciding on your meals, keep your salt and sugar intake low. Be more aware of how much sodium and sugar you are consuming for overall health.
- Use less dressings on your salads and foods. Enjoy the natural flavours.
- Slow down while you're eating, and enjoy the real taste of your food.
- Be reasonable in regard to portion size. Follow the guidelines on page 42.

- When you feel full, stop eating. When your body has had enough, it will let you know. Listen to your body and the messages it's sending.
- Don't go grocery shopping on an empty stomach. Create a shopping list before you go and stick to it. This will help to avoid adding foods to your cart that you don't need or shouldn't eat.
- Purchase foods that help you lose weight rather than gain it, following Izzy's Eating Plan guidelines.
- Get outside your comfort zone. Increase your meal options and try foods you've never tried before.
- Feel great about what's in your shopping cart.
- Get outside to enjoy the fresh air.
- Be more physically active in your daily routine. Even small changes can make a big difference.
- Exercise regularly to boost weight loss.
- Take your lunch to work.
- When eating out, stay within Izzy's Eating Plan as much as possible. Use the guidelines to make healthier, wiser choices.
- Get enough sleep.
- Reduce alcohol consumption.

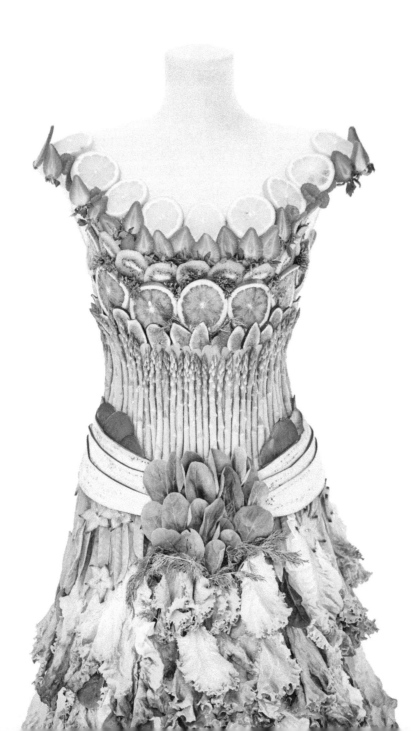

MENOPAUSE: A NOTE TO WOMEN APPROACHING OR BEYOND THE AGE OF 50

I wanted to include some information on menopause, which I am currently going through... (ugh). Just before its onset, I did my due diligence by doing some research.

During this time in a woman's life, there is a lot going on internally. By simply being aware of what's happening to your body and all of it's changes, you can try to limit its effects. Many women are not aware that weight gain will almost always happen during menopause if they don't make changes to their diet. This is partly because your body no longer requires as many calories as when you were still menstruating. My eating plan will not only help you reduce your calories, but make sure the ones you are consuming are the right ones to maintain a healthy weight.

CHAPTER 4

LIFESTYLE CHOICES
– GET OUTSIDE!

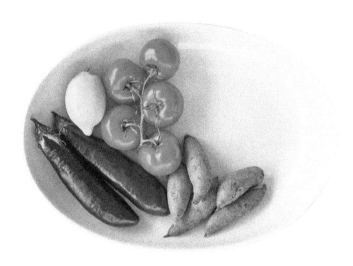

LIFESTYLE CHOICES
– GET OUTSIDE!

Have you ever gotten a one year gym membership, with the best intentions to workout regularly, only to find you've used it 2-3 times within that year? I've got my hand up! I once joined a gym located on my way home from work. "That's super convenient", I thought, "I'll be able to go all the time!". I think I went twice. Exercising was always something I've had a hard time committing to. It wasn't until I started to respect my body and take care of it, that I felt I was ready for such a commitment. I didn't want to get another gym membership knowing I wouldn't use it regularly. I used to enjoy jogging when I was younger, but had to stop due to the impact on my knees. Instead, I chose walking for my activity of choice. Not a Sunday stroll kind of walk, but the kind of walk where you're late for an appointment. Walking that gets your heart rate up and makes you break a sweat. Yup... walking. It's free, doesn't require special clothing or equipment, is low impact and right outside your door (super easy to get to!). To further increase my workout, I pick routes in my neighbourhood that have some hills. Generally, my walks last for 30 minutes to an hour, allowing me to walk up to 5km. This is 'me time'. I take this time to think through stuff clouding my head, or don't think at all. Sometimes I listen to music, other times I enjoy the silence. Just getting outside and breathing fresh air has amazing benefits, even if your physical abilities or time is limited (20 minutes a day is a great start!). Give yourself 'me time' daily, and remember to get outside, breathe deep, unwind and relax.

You might be the type of person that doesn't need a push to exercise, so for you, you need no motivation from me. For those that do need a little nudge, here are some simple ways to get yourself moving:

- Wake up each morning with simple stretches to start the day and get your body moving.
- Start walking/wheeling regularly, or start a new physical activity.
- If possible, take the stairs instead of elevators.
- Get on or off the bus 1 or 2 stops before your destination and walk/wheel the rest.
- Walk/wheel to or from your destination if possible.
- Shop locally so you don't need your car.
- When driving, park further away from the entrance.
- Take on a new sport or hobby for fun.
- Get a walking/wheeling or workout buddy.
- Take yoga or other exercise classes.
- Walk your dog or a friend's.

- Go for a stroll after dinner to help with your digestion and allow for a better night's sleep.

It's important for overall health to get enough sleep which also helps maintain an ideal weight. Sleep deprivation affects us negatively in many ways, mentally and physically, and can contribute to weight gain.

CHAPTER 5

IZZY'S EATING PLAN: SO EXCITED TO SHARE!

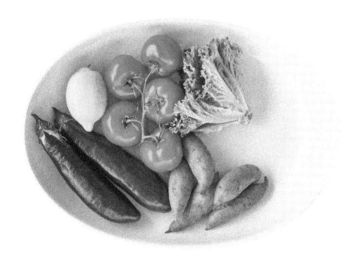

IZZY'S EATING PLAN: SO EXCITED TO SHARE!

Outlined here is Izzy's Eating Plan! Simply put, it's about eating the right foods together that won't spike blood sugar and insulin levels thus reducing fat production. Following the simple guidelines around food makes maintaining my plan super easy.

Izzy's Eating Plan is about giving your body what it needs to stay healthy, function properly and feel awesome after every meal and every snack. It's about giving yourself the right foods to fuel your body, feel full and satisfied. These foods will positively affect you by improving other parts of your body too (heart, skin, bones and brain), while providing nutrients throughout the day. It's a 'win-win' combination.

Izzy's Eating Plan Guidelines:

Before we get into the details of my eating plan, I quickly want to discuss portion size. For proteins, your serving size should be roughly the size of your palm (not including your thumb or your fingers). With most other foods, a handful or two is often enough. Use cheeses in moderation. Make common sense the rule. If you are trying to lose weight, keep your portion sizes reasonable and stop eating when you are full.

The instructions around this plan are as simple as being able to count to 2. Yup, it's that simple.

The foods listed here have been divided into groups. Group 0, 1 and 2. These are foods that are readily available from your local grocery store. In fact, you are likely eating many of these foods already. On my plan, the difference will be what foods you choose to eat together at each individual meal or snack. Allow me to explain.

Each meal you eat throughout the day, including snacks, should not exceed a total of 2. This is determined by adding together the assigned group number of each food on your plate. It will become second nature as you get used to what foods can and cannot be eaten together.

Understanding the Food Groups:

Described below are the Food Groups and how they work during meal planning. It will become easier to create your meals, as you become more familiar with the Food Groups. For this reason, I have included some examples, good and bad, to help guide you.

You will find these examples on page 52, after the Food Group Charts.

Group 0: You can eat as many of these foods as you want, and they can be freely combined at each meal or snack. When you fill your plate with Group 0 foods, you can feel good knowing there will only be a positive impact on your body. Because these foods take longer to digest, you will feel full and satisfied longer. Just make sure that what you choose to eat with them, from Groups 1 or 2, does not add up to more than 2.

Group 1: Unlike Group 0, you can have a maximum of two Group 1 foods at each meal or snack. Group 1 foods can be eaten with any amount of foods from Group 0, however, you cannot combine any foods from Group 2. Doing so will bring your plate total to 3 which results in too many carbohydrates for one meal or snack, when eaten at the same time. Excessive carbohydrate consumption in a single meal can lead to weight gain.

Group 2: Foods in Group 2 are richer in carbohydrates or have a higher fat content. That being said, these foods can only be eaten with foods from Group 0. Combining Group 0 foods to the richer Group 2 foods helps balance blood sugar levels, which is one of the important keys to weight loss and maintaining a healthy weight.

In a super simple way, this system allows you to always be in control of your weight. Yup... in control!

Izzy's Eating Plan and Food Group Chart

GROUP 0

MEAT & POULTRY (ALL SELECTIONS CONTAIN PROTEIN)
- Chicken
- Rabbit
- Turkey

FISH (ALL SELECTIONS CONTAIN PROTEIN)
- Cod
- Flounder
- Haddock
- Mahi Mahi
- Orange Roughy
- Red Snapper
- Sole

SHELLFISH (ALL SELECTIONS CONTAIN PROTEIN)
- Calamari
- Clams
- Crab
- Lobster
- Mussels
- Oysters
- Scallops
- Shrimp

LEGUMES (ALL SELECTIONS CONTAIN PROTEIN)

- Tofu/Tempeh

VEGETABLES

- Artichokes
- Arugula
- Asparagus
- Bell Peppers
- Broccoli
- Brussels Sprouts
- Cabbage/Sauerkraut
- Cauliflower
- Celery
- Collard Greens
- Cucumbers
- Eggplant
- Garlic
- Green Beans
- Hearts of Palm
- Kale
- Mushrooms
- Parsley
- Romaine Lettuce
- Snap Peas
- Snow Peas
- Spinach
- Swiss Chard
- Watercress
- Zucchini

DRINKS & LIQUIDS

- Coffee - black, organic if possible, 2 cups/ day max.
- Green Tea
- Herbal Tea
- Water with Fresh Lemon
- Chicken Stock - low sodium
- Beef Stock - low sodium
- Vegetable Stock - low sodium

GROUP 1

MEAT & POULTRY (ALL SELECTIONS CONTAIN PROTEIN)

- Beef
- Lamb

FISH (ALL SELECTIONS CONTAIN PROTEIN)

- Tilapia
- Trout

DAIRY (ALL SELECTIONS CONTAIN PROTEIN)

- Cottage Cheese
- Feta Cheese
- Goat Cheese
- Plain Greek Yogurt
- Ricotta Cheese
- Unsweetened Almond Milk

VEGETABLES

- Beets

- Butternut Squash
- Carrots
- Onions
- Spaghetti Squash

LEGUMES/LENTILS (ALL SELECTIONS CONTAIN PROTEIN)

- Black Beans
- Chickpeas/Hummus
- Green Peas
- Kidney Beans
- Mung Beans
- Navy Beans
- Red/Yellow/Green Lentils
- Romano Beans

FRUITS

- Apples
- Apricots
- Blackberries
- Blueberries
- Cherries
- Dates
- Grapefruit
- Lemons
- Limes
- Nectarines
- Olives
- Oranges
- Peaches
- Pears
- Plums

- Prunes
- Raspberries
- Strawberries
- Tangerines
- Tomatoes
- Watermelon

DRINKS
- Diluted Fruit Juice - 1/4 juice, 3/4 water

GROUP 2

MEAT & POULTRY (ALL SELECTIONS CONTAIN PROTEIN)
- Duck
- Goose
- Pork
- Prosciutto - nitrate free recommended
- Salami - nitrate free recommended
- 2 Eggs - prepared w/o fat

FISH (ALL SELECTIONS CONTAIN PROTEIN)
- Albacore Tuna
- Arctic Char
- Halibut
- Herring
- Mackerel
- Sardines
- Swordfish
- Wild Salmon

DAIRY (ALL SELECTIONS CONTAIN PROTEIN)
- Brie Cheese
- Cheddar Cheese
- Mozzarella Cheese
- Parmesan Cheese

GRAINS AND SEEDS
- Brown Rice
- Couscous
- Homemade Bran or Oatmeal Muffin
- Oats/Oatmeal - rolled or steel cut
- Popcorn - plain
- Quinoa (contains protein)
- Whole Grain Bread
- Whole Grain Pasta (for example, spelt or kamut)

VEGETABLES
- Bean Sprouts
- Corn - non GMO recommended
- Pumpkin
- Sweet Potatoes

FRUITS
- Avocado
- Bananas
- Coconut
- Grapes
- Mango
- Melons (Cantaloupe, Honeydew)
- Papaya
- Pineapple

DESSERTS
- Dark Chocolate - 70% Cacao or more
- Fruit Sorbets
- Honey
- Unsweetened Coconut Ice Cream

How we prepare our foods, as well as the dressings and sauces we add, can often make our meals heavy. When following my eating plan, the addition of heavy dressings and sauces will exceed the allowance of 2 for any meal or snack.

For salads, if you must use a dressing, try some fresh lemon juice or vinegars, such as Balsamic or flavoured vinegars Raspberry or Pomegranate. These options help reduce calories normally found in prepared salad dressings, yet adds loads of flavour. Another option is to add some shredded cheese to your salad, which also serves as a protein for your meal.

It is not recommended to use low-fat products, or any food labeled "low-fat", "low-calorie" or "diet" for that matter. Not only can "low-fat" labels lead to over eating, these products often have increased amounts of trans fats, sugar, salt and other additives, making them actually more harmful than healthful. We need fats to survive, and we need to make sure we're consuming healthy fats. Essential fatty acids help your body absorb certain vitamins, contributing to over all health, and reduce the risk of developing heart disease.

When cooking or grilling, use butter or coconut oil in moderation. Low-sodium soup stocks can also be used. Try some soup stock as an alternative to water when making brown rice or quinoa, for a different flavour. Herbs and spices can be used freely.

Get creative while learning healthier ways to prepare your food and enjoy your new way of eating!

Here are some good examples of well-balanced meals and snacks with food group combinations for a better understanding of how my eating plan works. Bad examples have also been included for some extra guidance.

Examples of what your meals could look like following Izzy's Eating Plan:

BREAKFAST:

Example #1
2x Egg Omelette - Group 1
Spinach - Group 0
Asparagus - Group 0
Feta Cheese - Group 1
Green Tea - Group 0
Total for meal: 1 + 0 + 0 + 1 + 0 = 2

Example #2
Unsweetened Greek Yogurt - 1
Blueberries - 1
Black Tea or Coffee - 0
Total for meal: 1 + 1 + 0 = 2

LUNCH:

Example #1
Spinach - 0
Celery - 0
Cucumber - 0
Bell Peppers - 0
Tomatoes - 1
Carrots - 1
Grilled Chicken - 0
Herbal Tea - 0
Total for meal: 0 + 0 + 0 + 0 + 1 + 1 + 0 + 0 = 2

Example #2
Hummus - 1
Carrots - 1
Celery - 0
Asparagus - 0
Cauliflower - 0
Lemon Water - 0
Total for meal: 1 + 1 + 0 + 0 + 0 + 0 = 2

DINNER:

Example #1
Sweet Potato - 2
Steamed Broccoli - 0
Steamed Cauliflower - 0
Steamed Asparagus - 0
Cod Fish - 0
Green Tea - 0
Total for meal: 2 + 0 + 0 + 0 + 0 + 0 = 2

Example #2
Kale - 0
Brussels Sprouts - 0
Zucchini - 0
Whole Grain Rice - 2
Tofu - 0
Water - 0
Total for meal: 0 + 0 + 0 + 2 + 0 + 0 = 2

The following are *bad* examples, where the totals add up to more than 2:

Example #1
Oatmeal - 2
Blueberries - 1
Strawberries - 1
Black Coffee or Tea - 0
Total for meal: 2 + 1 + 1 + 0 = 4

Example #2
Romaine Lettuce - 0
Celery - 0
Carrots - 1
Bell Peppers - 0
Tomatoes - 1
Chick Peas - 1
Turkey - 0
Total for meal: 0 + 0 + 1 + 0 + 1 + 1 + 0 = 3

Example #3
Brown Rice - 2
Steamed Green Beans - 0
Steamed Carrots - 1
Pork - 2
Apple - 1
Water with Lemon - 0
Total for meal: 2 + 0 + 1 + 2 + 1 + 0 = 6

Snacks can be eaten between main meals. Mid-morning and mid-afternoon are ideal times. I like to have an apple for one of my snacks, as they are great cleansers, filling and yummy. Any fruits from Groups 1 or 2 are a good choice. Another good option to have on hand is cut veggies. Eat them alone, or with some hummus. Just be sure to keep your snacks light, and their total should not add up to more than 2 – the same rules apply to snacks as main meals.

As you are getting started on Izzy's Eating Plan, here are some important reminders:

- Proteins take longer to digest allowing for a full and satisfied feeling. Try to include protein at each main meal.
- Keep hydrated throughout the day with water and other fluids recommended on the plan.
- Have healthy snacks on hand to fuel your body mid-morning and mid-afternoon.
- Make the switch from white breads, white pastas and white rice to whole grain breads, whole grain pastas and brown rice. They're healthier, tastier and have more fibre to keep you full longer.
- Get creative with your cooking and try foods or meals you've never tried before.
- When making meals, cook a bit extra to use for lunches or meals later in the week. It will save you time and money!
- Eat fresh foods over pre-packaged or processed.
- When eating out, it may be difficult to stay within the limit of '2', so try to make healthier, lighter choices as best you can.
- Eat slowly and chew your food well. Savour the flavour.
- Be aware of portion size and stop eating when you are full.
- Reduce or eliminate the salt and sugar you add to your foods and drinks.

- Reduce alcohol consumption.
- Exercise regularly and keep active. Make a point to move your body every day.
- Get enough sleep.

Maintenance: Once You Get There... You CAN Stay There.

You've reached your goal weight!!! Yay!!!... now what? I've asked that same question when I would reach my goal on other diet plans. By this time, I was so over it and feeling deprived that I had no interest in a 'maintenance' program, figuring I didn't need it. I had reached my goal! Why would I need to still follow a diet? So... I went back to eating how I ate before, assuming my weight would not return, like I had trained my body to be resistant to fat. As I write this, I realize how silly that sounds. Obviously, if I go back to old eating habits, I'll go back to the weight I was... duh! But now, with this realization, there's no going back! Those days are over. Knowing what I know now gives me the strength to eat with intention. I don't even have to think about it, it's just how I roll these days. It makes me feel great making healthier choices at every meal. Every... single... solitary... meal... even my snacks.

Introducing Group 3

Once you've reached your goal weight, you need to maintain it. The maintenance part of my eating plan introduces a third Food Group to give you more variety and flexibility. Group 3. This group is higher in healthy fats and calories. The same rules apply, but with the addition of this group, your meals can now add up to 3. This gives you a bit more freedom with the options and combinations, but still keeps you on track.

Below is Group 3 of Izzy's Eating Plan.

GROUP 3

DELI MEATS (ALL SELECTIONS CONTAIN PROTEIN)
- Bacon - nitrate free recommended
- Patés

GRAINS
- Whole Grain Bagels
- Whole Grain Crackers
- Croissants
- Granola

DAIRY
- Butter
- Cream

NUTS & SEEDS (ALL SELECTIONS CONTAIN PROTEIN)

- Almond Butter
- Almonds
- Brazil Nuts
- Cashews
- Pumpkin Seeds
- Sesame Seeds
- Sunflower Seeds
- Walnuts

VEGETABLES

- White Potatoes

FRUITS

- Dried Apples
- Dried Apricots
- Dried Cranberries
- Raisins

DESSERTS

- Cheesecake (contains protein)
- Flour-free Chocolate Cake
- Fruit Flan
- Fruit Pie
- Pure Jam

Here are a couple of examples including Food Group 3:

BREAKFAST:

Oatmeal - 2
Blueberries - 1
Black Tea or Coffee - 0
Total for meal: 2 + 1 + 0 = 3

LUNCH:

Couscous - 2
Black Beans - 1
Bell Peppers - 0
Cucumbers - 0
Parsley - 0
Green Tea - 0
Total for meal: 2 + 1 + 0 + 0 + 0 + 0 = 3

DINNER:

Brown Rice - 2
Grilled Beef - 1
Grilled Bell Peppers - 0
Grilled Zucchini - 0
Water w/Lemon - 0
Total for meal: 2 + 1 + 0 + 0 + 0 = 3

Meals prepared over a total of 3, would not be following the guidelines of the maintenance plan.

HEALTHY DIET:

During the process of digestion, after consuming healthy complex carbohydrate foods (high fibre foods), sugars from these foods slowly enter the blood stream. The hormone insulin is then released more gradually from our pancreas to help move sugars from our blood, into our cells so they can be utilized as energy. Eating a consistent healthy well balanced diet will result in maintaining a healthy weight.

With Izzy's Eating Plan, we are consuming healthy, high fibre, nutrient dense foods that help keep blood sugar and insulin levels balanced throughout the day therefore, helping to maintain an ideal weight.

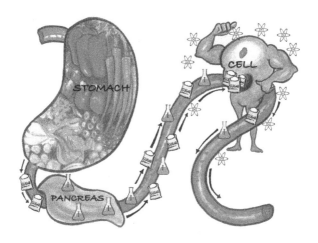

CHAPTER 6

FINDING NEW WAYS: LOOKING AT FOOD DIFFERENTLY

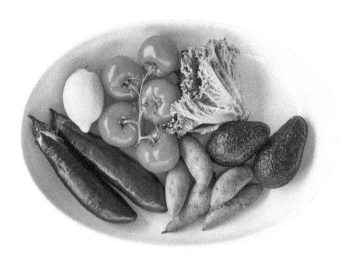

FINDING NEW WAYS: LOOKING AT FOOD DIFFERENTLY

Learn to reshape the way you eat. It is possible to cut out foods that you love eating and replace them with something else that's better for you. We all get stuck in our ways... and it IS possible to get unstuck.

As you get used to your new way of eating, you may find yourself no longer needing to eat foods you used to classify as 'staples'. For me, this was bread. I never thought it would be humanly possible to cut out bread, but now I eat very little of it. Because bread is in Group 2, I found it difficult to have with my meals the same way I used to, without exceeding a total of 2. When I felt my body needed a carbohydrate, I opted for brown rice or legumes, which turned out to be just as satisfying, kept me within my limit of 2 and also provided the essential complex carbohydrates I needed to fuel my body and brain. It made me realize that I do not need bread to be a happy and complete person.

During my weight loss stage, I created a salad, which I had on a regular basis, and started calling it my 'Power Salad'.

My Power Salad recipe is quite simple. It contains vegetables, with a protein, that focus on improving the areas of the body that are highlighted in this book: skin, bones, heart, brain, and overall cleansing. By looking at the lists of foods under each category, I put together several combinations, focusing on the areas I wanted to improve, while being mindful not to exceed my meal's total (2 when trying to lose weight, or 3 during maintenance). Having these Power Salads on a regular basis helped me reach my goals, not only with weight loss, but also with improving specific areas of my body. And, because the vegetable portion of the salad is raw, it gives my insides a regular workout and a good cleanse.

Here's an example of a typical Power Salad, keeping within a total of 2:

POWER SALAD:

Romaine Lettuce - 0
Spinach - 0
Asparagus - 0
Beets - 1
Carrots - 1
Celery - 0

Snap Peas - 0
Grilled Chicken/Tofu/Tempeh - 0
Total for meal: 0 + 0 + 0 + 1 + 1 + 0 + 0 + 0 = 2

Other options could include vegetables from the Group 0 list and one protein from Group 2. Any combination works. Just remember to keep within a maximum of 2 during weight loss, and 3 during maintenance.

Now I happily fuel my body with healthy food. I eat with intention. When I stray, I come right back, no guilt. It's easier now to find my way back because I know what to do. Instead of feeling lost and over-whelmed, I remind myself that I am in control. My actions create both my weight gain and my weight loss. No more 'going on a diet'... I just stick to my plan and my weight is maintained... simply. I say "simply" because eating this way makes me feel great, and I want to keep feeling great. It's easier for me to respect my body now that it's healthy and I will continue to treat it with respect for the rest of my life. I know what it took to get me where I am... I now want to stay here.

CHAPTER 7

AN APPLE A DAY

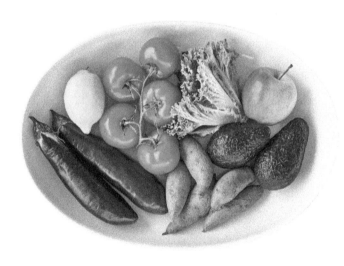

AN APPLE A DAY

We're busy people, living very busy lives. I know firsthand that eating healthy can be challenging. It's been that way for me in the past, but now, with my new attitude regarding food, it's really not that hard. There's been a shift in the way I look at and decide what foods I'm going to purchase and consume.

Sticking to this new way of eating will be life altering. You will change how you eat and how you think about food. You will find yourself being more conscious and critical of what you put into your body. It will make you realize that how you ate before did not get you to your optimal health and weight. You will feel better, both physically and mentally.

Become an inspiration to yourself and others. Reaching your goal weight, or even while on your way, you will begin to inspire your family, friends or coworkers without even trying. They will notice differences in you.

Following this eating plan opened my eyes. My new knowledge and understanding of food gave me the power to reach my optimal weight and keep it there. You too can have this power! WANT to make a change. Put your health and body FIRST. Be accountable for your food choices one meal at a time... starting right now!

Through unconscious consumption, we may be harming our bodies without realizing it. That is why there is no time to waste - we need to take action now. Negative and serious health issues are on the rise, and they are starting younger and younger. It is increasingly important as we age, to take care of ourselves now in order to have a healthier future. Remember the old saying, "An apple a day keeps the doctor away." This truthful statement should serve as a reminder to take food more seriously and to fuel our bodies with healthy foods. Prevention is better than a cure. You become what you eat, so eat well.

We are a product of the generations before us, just as they were a product of the generations before them. If we continue to eat unhealthily, future generations will suffer. They will be a direct result of our present actions. Take a moment to let this sink in. Our eating habits affect our lives AND those we create. Eating healthily and leading by example is the best thing we can do for ourselves, our children and future generations. Let's make our eating habits excellent ones and we can all move toward a healthier world and future.

This is not a diet, but an eating plan. One that you can easily follow now and for the rest of your life to maintain a healthy weight and better you.

With fashion design and outer beauty being the focus of my life's work, I'm now focusing on inner beauty, overall health and well-being.

Be good to yourself,

Izzy

ACKNOWLEDGEMENTS

I wanted to thank the following beautiful people for helping me with this book. Without their awesomeness, Izzy's Eating Plan would not be possible.

Thank you, Joanne Smith, from the bottom of my heart. Thank you for helping me make Izzy's Eating Plan a reality. Thank you for listening to me during the early days of understanding what changes my body was going through and agreeing that writing a book about it was actually a good idea. Thank you for validating my ideas and helping me share them through Izzy's Eating Plan. I am forever grateful.

Thank you, Bel Owen, for helping me organize my thoughts, way back when I started writing the book. I was all over the place and you managed to reel me in and put some order into my plan through your own genius and patience.

Thank you, Chris Chapman, for being one of my best friends and helping me add visuals to the book - to all my projects for that matter. Wrapping our heads around this one, was tough initially, but we did it. I love the cover - love, love, love! I love everything you've done for me and my career. You've made every piece timeless and I love you dearly for that.

Thank you, Peter Defreitas, for being who you are to me in life. Thank you for creating the illustrations for my book. This project was a far cry from a fashion illustration, but you nailed it. Your art is now a helpful tool to visualize what goes on inside us in a fun, simple to understand way. I love that you are a part of it.

Thank you, Rebecca Mezger, for helping me edit the book, helping me clean up my writing and stream line my thoughts. Anyone who knows me knows I can make a short story really long. This book took us out of our day to day routine and added a new feather to our caps.

Thank you, Jackie Shawn, for your mastery on the day of the shoot and every time I need it. Thank you for pulling out the beauty in all of us through your make-up and hair artistry. You are a beautiful soul.

Thank you, David Kerr, for creating our Behind the Scene videos. You captured on film, in such a beautiful way, what it took to make that crazy gown made of fresh fruits and veggies. Thank you too for all the bear hugs!

Thank you, Sage Dakota, for helping us with your Food Stylist creativity. Me being a novice at working with food in this way, you helped guide us in creating the gown with your tools and expertise.

Thank you, Vanessa Furtado, in helping me create Izzy's Eating Plan, both in book form and creating the website so I could share it with the world. Thank you for your patience with my requests - they seemed to be endless, I'm sure. The results in the end are exactly what I envisioned.

And last but not least, thank you, to Karl Zakss, for being my lovely assistant the day of our shoot creating the gown and more importantly in life. Thank you for putting up with me through thick and thin. Thank you for being my best friend.

9 781773 029696